Olfa Hammami
Asma Jelassi

Severe asthma exacerbations in children

Olfa Hammami
Asma Jelassi

Severe asthma exacerbations in children

Management

ScienciaScripts

Imprint

Any brand names and product names mentioned in this book are subject to trademark, brand or patent protection and are trademarks or registered trademarks of their respective holders. The use of brand names, product names, common names, trade names, product descriptions etc. even without a particular marking in this work is in no way to be construed to mean that such names may be regarded as unrestricted in respect of trademark and brand protection legislation and could thus be used by anyone.

Cover image: www.ingimage.com

This book is a translation from the original published under ISBN 978-620-6-71807-9.

Publisher:
Sciencia Scripts
is a trademark of
Dodo Books Indian Ocean Ltd. and OmniScriptum S.R.L publishing group

120 High Road, East Finchley, London, N2 9ED, United Kingdom
Str. Armeneasca 28/1, office 1, Chisinau MD-2012, Republic of Moldova, Europe
Printed at: see last page
ISBN: 978-620-8-18867-2

Copyright © Olfa Hammami, Asma Jelassi
Copyright © 2024 Dodo Books Indian Ocean Ltd. and OmniScriptum S.R.L publishing group

TABLE OF CONTENTS

Introduction

Asthma is one of the most common chronic diseases in children, and currently represents a major public health challenge worldwide. The condition affects 300 million people worldwide, including 30 million in Europe [1]. The most recent summaries of epidemiological data concerning asthma in France report a cumulative prevalence of asthma of over 10% in children aged over ten, while the current prevalence of asthma in adults is 6-7% [2]. The prevalence of asthma does not appear to be decreasing in France. Indeed, in some countries, no decrease in hospitalization rates has been observed in children in recent years [3]. For the under-15s, the frequency of asthma was 13% according to a national survey carried out in Tunisia in 1985 [4].

The prevalence of asthma currently affects 10% of children in Tunisia [4]. Although similarities can be observed between adult and childhood asthma, the paediatric population presents specific characteristics, particularly with regard to exacerbations.

An exacerbation is defined as persistent respiratory symptoms lasting more than 24 hours, regardless of whether the onset is gradual or abrupt, and requiring a change in treatment [2].

A severe exacerbation of asthma (SEA) is characterized by an alteration in the patient's usual state of health, as well as an unresponsiveness to well-administered medical treatment that can be life-threatening and requires urgent treatment.

In France, mortality associated with asthma exacerbations is relatively low [2]. In Brazil, the incidence of mortality was 0.21 per 100,000 people with asthma in 2014 [5]. In Mexico, the mortality rate was 0.36% [5]. To date, mortality data for asthmatic children in Tunisia are limited.

It is therefore imperative to identify children at risk of severe asthma exacerbations. Early management of these cases is crucial, to prevent recourse to mechanical ventilation and improve the overall prognosis of the disease.

We conducted a retrospective, longitudinal and descriptive study in the pediatrics department of Bizerte University Hospital.

This study included all children under 15 years of age hospitalized for severe asthma exacerbations over a period of 1 year and 6 months, from January 1, 2022 to June 30, 2023.

The aim of our study was to investigate the clinical, para-clinical, therapeutic and evolutionary characteristics of patients hospitalized for ESA in a general pediatric ward.

Methods

1. The type of study :

This is a retrospective, longitudinal and descriptive study, conducted within the pediatrics department at Bizerte University Hospital.

This study included all children under 15 years of age hospitalized for severe asthma exacerbations during a period of 1 year and 6 months from January 1, 2022 to June 30, 2023.

2. The patients

2-1- Inclusion criteria :

Children under 15 years of age were included, known to be asthmatic or not, and having presented a severe asthma exacerbation (SEA), in the pediatrics department of the University Hospital of Bizerte.

2-2- Criteria for non-inclusion :

Patients hospitalized for respiratory distress with a diagnosis other than severe asthma exacerbation (SEA) were not included.

2-3- Exclusion criteria :

Mild to moderate asthma exacerbations were excluded.

3. Definitions :

- An exacerbation is defined as persistent respiratory symptoms lasting more than 24 hours, regardless of whether the onset is gradual or abrupt, and requiring a change in treatment [2].
- Severe asthma exacerbation (SAE) is defined as a change in the patient's usual condition, which is also unresponsive to well-conducted medical treatment, may be life-

threatening and requires urgent treatment [2].

• Severe respiratory distress has been defined as significant polypnoea accompanied by clear signs of respiratory struggle, with or without hypoxia (Pulse Oxygen Saturation (SpO2) ≤ to 94% on room air) [6].

4. **Methods :**

Data were collected from hospitalization records, and children were selected during the study period.

4-1- Data collection :

A pre-established form was completed for all children with asthma. Data collected included (Appendix 1):

- Socio-demographic characteristics: age, gender, comorbidity, age, urban or rural origin, family atopy.

- The evolution of asthmatic disease.

- The current ESA phase involves :

o Triggering factors.
o Clinical respiratory signs: respiratory rate, O2 saturation SpO2, SpO2/FiO2 ratio,
o Gasometric data, neurological signs and cardiovascular signs.

- Management includes respiratory assistance techniques, the administration of short-acting bronchodilators (SADBs) and the route used, the use of corticosteroids and the administration of magnesium sulfate.

- Evolution:

o Duration of hospitalization (days).
o Duration of oxygen therapy.
o Ventilatory complications (atelectasis, intra-thoracic gas effusion),
o Bacterial or viral superinfection,
o Healthcare-associated infections.
o Death rate.

4-2- Valuation methods :

According to the criteria defined by GINA 2021, the level of asthma control was assessed (Appendix 2) [1], as was the level of previous treatment (Appendix 3) [1].

5. Bibliographic research :

To carry out our bibliographic search, we consulted the following search engines: Pubmed - Science direct.

References were entered and organized using ZOTERO

Key words: "Child", "asthma attack", "exacerbation of disease", "taking charge".

6. Ethical considerations :

We declare that there are no conflicts of interest in this work.

Patient data sheets were kept anonymous.

Results

1- The impact :

During the study period, 3751 children were hospitalized on the pediatric ward.
of the University Hospital of Bizerte.
Thirty patients were admitted for ESA, representing 0.7% of the total hospitalized
population.

The incidence was 0.7 new cases of ESA/100 hospitalizations in the pediatric ward.

2- Socio-demographic characteristics :

2-1- Age :

The mean age of patients was 47±30 months, with extremes ranging from 10.8 to 132
months.

The age range >3 years is the most represented in our series (n=18): 13 patients
aged between 3 and 6 years and five patients aged over 6 years.

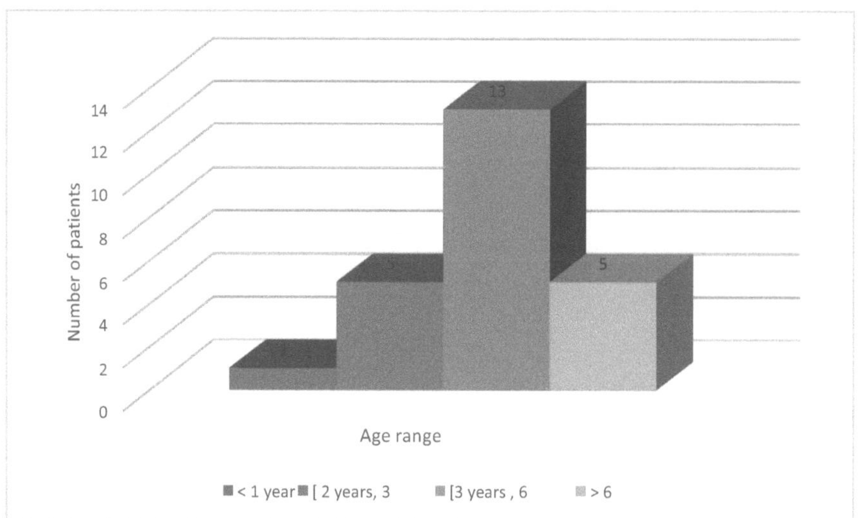

Figure 1: Distribution of hospitalized patients by age.

2-2- Sex :

The study population comprised 15 boys (50%) and 15 girls (50%). The gender ratio (M/F) was 1.

2-3- The month of hospitalization :

Over the month of April, the admission rate of patients hospitalized for severe asthma exacerbations, peaked at 20%.

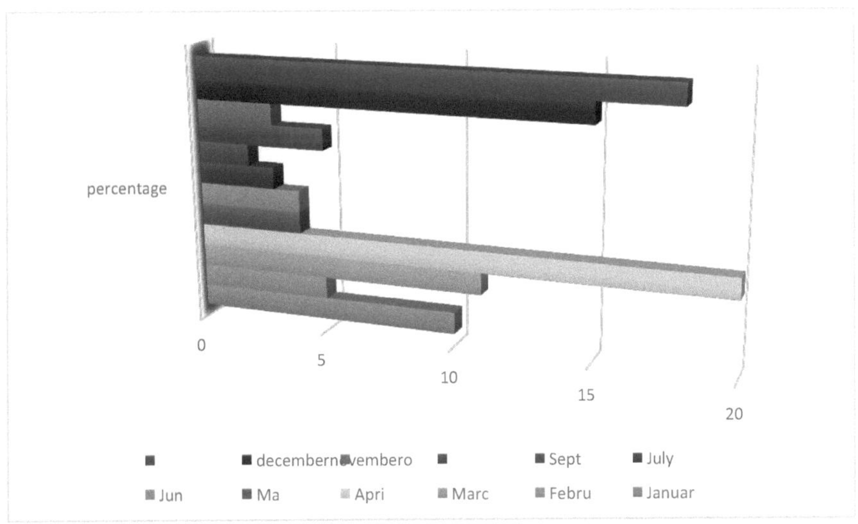

Figure 2: Distribution of patients by month of admission.

2-4- Comorbidities and hospitalization history :

Thirteen of our patients (43%) had concomitant allergic manifestations (2 cases of atopic dermatitis, 7 cases of allergic rhinitis and 4 cases of allergic conjunctivitis), eight patients (26%) had iron-deficiency anemia and one patient (3%) was overweight.

Eighteen patients (60%) were hospitalized for the first time. The remaining twelve patients (40%) had previous hospitalizations: ten for acute bronchiolitis and two for other reasons (hives, poisoning).

2-5-Environment :

Passive smoking was observed in 20 children (66%). However, the presence of pets was noted in 9 patients (30%). Twenty-three patients (76%) were exposed to humidity. Regarding habitat, a rural environment was reported in 4 patients (13%).

3- The evolution of asthmatic disease :

3-1- Atopy :

3-1-1- Familial atopy :

Familial atopy was detected on the parental side in 14 cases (46%): ten cases were linked to allergic asthma and four to allergic rhinitis.

Nine of our patients had a history of asthma in their siblings.

3-1-2- Personal atopy :

The history revealed allergic manifestations associated with asthma in 13 cases (43%): atopic dermatitis in 2 cases, allergic rhinitis in 7 cases and allergic conjunctivitis in 4 cases.

3-2- Age at diagnosis of asthma :

Twenty patients (66%) were diagnosed at the time of ESA, with a mean age of 47 ±30 months (10-132 months). Ten patients (33%) were labelled asthmatic, with a mean age of 11 ±13 months and extremes of 1-48 months.

3-3- Asthma management :

3-3-1- Medical follow-up :

➢ **The attending physician :**

Four of our patients were followed by an outpatient pediatrician, four by a hospital pediatrician and two by an adult outpatient pulmonologist.

➢ **Follow-up health structure :**

A third of known asthmatics were on disease-modifying therapy with regular follow-up.

Forty percent were monitored by an independent practitioner, 30% in a university hospital and 30% in a health facility.

3-3-2- Treatment received and compliance :

The ten children with known asthma were undergoing background treatment and were distributed as follows:

✓   45% were on on-demand short-acting bronchodilators
(Level 1).
✓   55% were on low-dose inhaled corticosteroids and bronchodilators
short-acting on-demand (Level 2).

Nine of these patients (90%) had partial asthma control with poor compliance, two of whom (20%) did not use the inhalation chamber.

3-4- Level of asthma control :

3-4-1- History of ESA and previous hospitalizations :

Six patients (60%) had a previous hospitalization for asthma exacerbation. Of these, five patients (83%) were admitted within the 4 months preceding the onset of the severe asthma exacerbation.

3-4-2- Classification according to level of asthma control :

Of the 10 children on background asthma treatment, 8 had uncontrolled asthma and 2 had partially controlled asthma over the last 4 weeks.

Four of our patients (13%) were truant from school and nine (30%) had aregular sporting activity.

4- Triggers and management of severe asthma exacerbations :

4-1- Triggering factors :

The triggers found are listed in Figure 3, with the most common being are viral infection, followed by pollution:

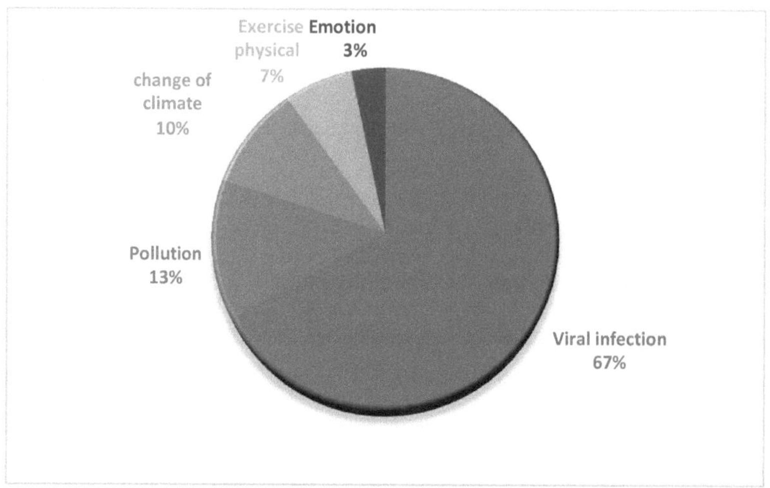

Figure 3: Triggers for ESA in our patients

4-2- Home treatment :

Eleven patients (36%) used inhaled short-acting bronchodilators. Ten patients (33%) received an oral corticosteroid dose of 1 mg/kg.

4-3- Hospitalization time :

The average hospital stay was 13 ± 11 hours. The minimum delay was 1 hour and the maximum 49 hours.

5- **Clinical signs :**

5-1- Body mass index (BMI) :

In our patients, the mean body mass index was 18±2 kg/m2 with values ranging from 14 to 26. Three of our patients were obese, with a BMI exceeding 97ème percentile.

5-2- Temperature :

Fever was noted in 17 patients (56%).
on admission was 37±0.8 (35.5-39.4).

5-3- Respiratory signs :

The mean respiratory rate was 52 ±10 cycles/minute, with extremes between 40 and 78. Sixty percent showed signs of intense struggle, 20% were in the exhaustion stage and a further 20% had moderate signs of struggle. Seventeen children were cyanotic and covered in sweat (56%).

Mean oxygen saturation (SpO2) was approximately 91±2% (82-95) in air.
ambient.

Ten patients had orthopnea (33%) and fourteen patients (46%) had slurred speech. Subcutaneous emphysema was observed in 3 patients (10%).

On pulmonary auscultation, we observed sibilants in 29 cases (96%) and auscultatory silence in 1 case (3%).

5-4- Cardiovascular signs :

The mean heart rate was 170 ±24 beats per minute, with extremes from 104 to 212. Four of our patients presented with shock on admission.

5-5- Neurological signs :

Consciousness was preserved in the majority of cases (70%). Neurological disorders were present in nine patients (30%), with agitation in six (20%) and confusion in three (10%), with GCS between 13 and 14/15.

13

5-6- Moisture status :

Two infants showed signs of mild dehydration.

6-   Additional tests :

6-1- Initial gasometry :

All patients had gas measurements, mean pH 7.3 (7.2-7.4). Mean PaO2 was 82 ±5 mm Hg (70-90). Mean PaCO2 was 36

±8 mmHg (22-52). Capnia exceeded 45mmHg in 6 children (20%) and was below 35mmHg in 15 children (50%).

Five of our patients showed respiratory acidosis (16%), respiratory alkalosis in 10 patients (33%) and metabolic acidosis in two patients.

6-2- Inflammatory assessment :

-    **Blood count :**

Mean hemoglobin was 11 ±1 g/dl, ranging from 10 to 13 g/dl. White blood cell count above 15,000/mm3 was noted in 13 children (43%). The mean eosinophil count was 661 ±174, ranging from 400 to 1200. Thrombocytopenia was not observed.

-    **C-reactive protein (CRP) :**

Performed in the presence of suspected bronchial superinfection, the mean CRP level was 46 ±95 mg/l, ranging from 2 to 500 mg/l. CRP above 50mg/l was observed in 5 patients.

6-3- Blood ionogram :

Hypokalemia was observed in 2 cases (6%) and hyponatremia in three cases (10%).

6-4- Microbiological tests :

Two patients had positive blood cultures. The germ isolated was multisensitive Streptococcus pneumoniae.

6-5- Chest X-ray :

All patients had bilateral pulmonary distension. It was associated with atelectasis in 6 cases (20%), a pneumomediastinum in 4 cases (13%), an alveolar focus in 8 cases (26%) and a pneumothorax in 1 case (3%) (figure4).

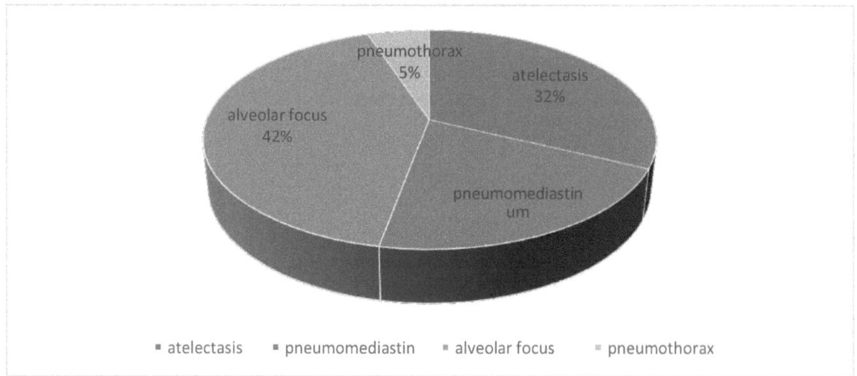

Figure 4: Radiological findings in our patients in addition to thoracic distension

7- **Therapeutic management :**

7-1- Short-acting bronchodilators :

- Terbutaline nebulizations:

Patients received nebulizations of terbutaline at a dose of 0.15mg/kg/nebulization every 15 to 20 minutes for the first hour, then every 4 hours.

- Ipratropium bromide nebulizations (Atrovent) :

Twenty-seven patients (90%) received nebulizations of inhaled anticholinergics, discontinuously in all patients. The dose used was 0.25mg/nebulization/8h.

7-2- Corticoids :

All our patients received intravenous corticosteroids. Methylprednisolone (Solumedrol) was the drug of choice, with a bolus dose of 2mg/kg, followed by 2mg/kg/day divided into 4 doses.

7-3- Magnesium sulfate :

Magnesium sulfate was administered in 70% of cases (21 patients). The dose used was 50mg/kg over 20 minutes. The average time taken to administer magnesium sulfate was 1 hour, ranging from 0 to 2 hours. A second dose was used in ten patients.

7-4- Ventilatory assistance :

- **Conventional oxygen therapy :**

Twenty-five patients (83%) received oxygen therapy via single nasal cannula or single mask.

- **Non-invasive ventilation (NIV) :**

High-flow oxygen therapy (HFO) was used in 5 patients (16%) with an average flow rate of 18 ±5 liters per minute, ranging from 7 to 35 liters per minute. For each patient, the flow rate corresponded to 2-3 l/kg/min. The mean duration of OHD was 38 ±35 hours, ranging from 1 to 190 hours.

- **Mechanical ventilation :**

None of our patients has used this technique.

7-5- Hemodynamic support :

Hemodynamic support was required in four patients. Two patients required vascular filling, and only two required vasoactive drugs. The molecules used were : Noradrenaline for 2 patients, in combination with adrenaline for 1.

The average duration of drug maintenance was 41 hours, ranging from 29 to 48 hours.

7-6- Antibiotic treatment :

Nineteen patients (63%) received antibiotic therapy. Ampicillin, cefotaxime and macrolides were the molecules used in our study.

Table I shows the distribution of patients hospitalized for severe exacerbation. asthma, depending on the antibiotic treatment prescribed.

Table I: Distribution of patients according to antibiotic treatment prescribed

AntibioticsNumberPercentage

Antibiotics	Number	Percentage
Ampicillin	12	40%
Cefotaxime	3	10%
Ampicillin+macrolides	2	6%
Cefotaxime+ macrolides	2	6%

Bacteremia was only proven by two blood cultures. The germ was multisensitive Streptococcus pneumoniae.

8- **Short-term trends :**

The average hospital stay was 4 ±1 days, ranging from 2 to 6 days. Twenty-four of our patients (80%) developed complications during their stay.

However, all patients had a favorable outcome.

8-1- Complications :

8-1-1- Complications related to ESA :

In our study, we noted the occurrence of pneumothorax in 1 case, pneumo mediastinum in 4 cases, atelectasis in 6 cases and hyponatremia in 3 cases.

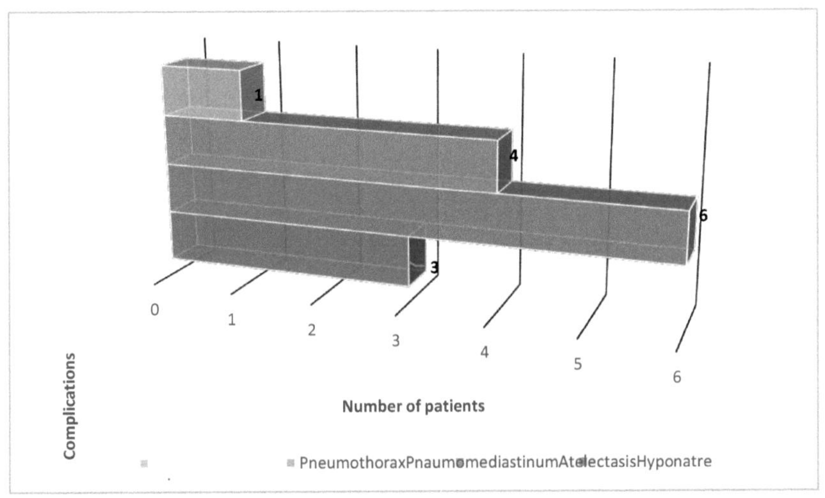

Figure 5: Distribution of complications associated with severe asthma exacerbations in our patients.

8-1-2- Treatment-related complications :

In our study, hyperglycemia occurred in 8 cases, and hypokalemia
in 2 cases. There were no cases of healthcare-associated infection or hypertension.

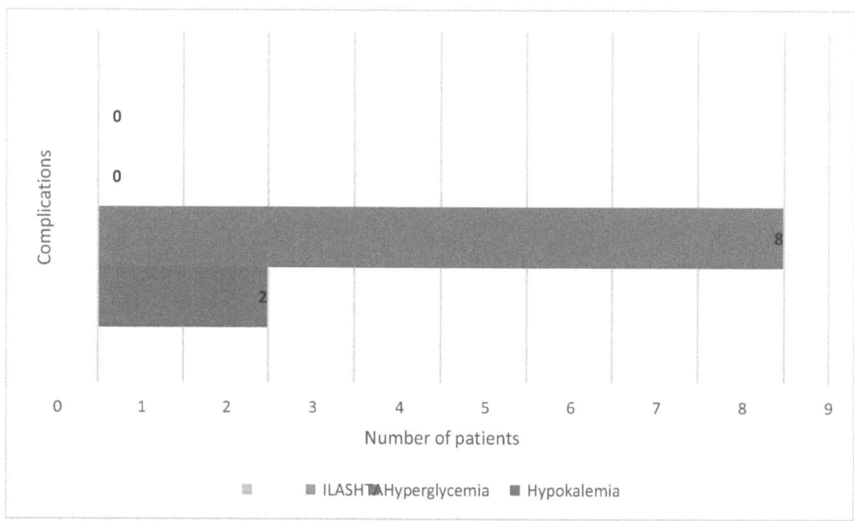

Figure 6: Summary diagram of observed treatment-related complications.

8-2- Mortality :

No fatalities were reported.

Discussion

1. Main results :

The main results obtained in our study showed a hospital incidence of ESA of 0.7 new cases/100 hospitalizations in the pediatric department. The mean age of our patients was 47 months ±3 (10-132 months) and the gender ratio was 1. Comorbidity was found in 73% of cases. Admissions peaked in April (20%). Thirteen patients (43%) had associated allergic manifestations, and none had a food allergy. Ten patients (33%) were known asthmatics. Six patients (60%) had been previously hospitalized for asthma exacerbation. The average hospital stay was 13 ±11 hours (1-48 hours). Prior to hospitalization, inhaled BDCAs were administered in 11 patients (36%). Oral corticosteroids were administered in ten patients (33%) at a dose of 1 mg/kg, prescribed at home.

Clinical examination on admission showed a mean respiratory rate of 52
±10 cycles/minute (40-78), mean SpO2 91±2% (82-95) on room air. Sixty percent of our patients had intense signs of struggle, 20% were in the exhaustion stage and 20% had moderate signs of struggle. Seventeen children were cyanotic and covered in sweat (56%). Pulmonary auscultation revealed auscultatory silence in 1 case (3%). Slurred speech was noted in fourteen patients (46%). Only one patient was in shock. Neurologically, 30% of our patients had consciousness disorders. For arterial gasometry, the mean pH was 7.3 (7.2-7.4) and the mean capnia was 36 ±8 mm Hg (22-52).

Hyponatremia was observed in three cases (10%). Hypokalemia was noted in 2 cases (6.6%).

Hyperleukocytosis was observed in 13 children (43%).   CRP above 50mg/l was observed in 5 patients.

Ventilatory disorders were noted in 36% of cases, and bilateral pulmonary distension in all patients was objectified on chest x-ray.

Therapeutically, all our patients received terbutaline nebulizations every 15 to 20 minutes for the first hour. Nebulizations of inhaled anticholinergics were administered in 27 patients (90%). From

Intravenous corticosteroids (methylprednisolone) were administered to all our patients. Magnesium sulfate was administered to 21 children (70%).

Conventional oxygen therapy was required in 83% of cases. High-flow oxygen therapy (HFO) was used in 5 patients (16%). None of our patients were intubated.

Seventeen patients (56%) received antibiotic therapy on clinical grounds. Bacterial co-infection was confirmed in only two patients. Complications were mainly ventilatory disorders such as atelectasis and hyperglycemia. No deaths were reported.

I. Strengths and limitations of the work :

1. Strengths of our study :

To the best of our knowledge, our study is one of the first nationwide to investigate ESA in a general paediatric ward. Our results alargely consistent with the literature.

2. Limitations of our work :

The retrospective nature of the study did not allow us to determine the risk factors for the occurrence of ESA. This is reflected in the information bias that accompanies retrospective studies

The pediatrics department at Bizerte University Hospital is not an intensive care unit, and does not have artificial ventilation facilities or a technical platform for protected bacteriological sampling.

II. **Socio-demographic characteristics :**

1- Incidence :

In our series, the incidence was 0.7 new cases of ESA/100 hospitalizations in the pediatric ward. A higher average incidence of 2 new cases/year/100 hospitalizations was reported in a study carried out in Spain in a university hospital, which caters for 200,000 children aged 0-14 years [7].

2- Age :

In our series, the majority of children were over 3 years of age, representing 60% of the sample. According to a study carried out in France, almost half of hospital admissions were in children aged 3 to 5 years [8]. The small size of the airways, which explains the lower threshold for onset of respiratory distress, and the frequency of viral respiratory infections may explain the increased risk of exacerbations in young asthmatic children [8].

3- Genre :

A predominance of males has been noted in several previous studies [9- 11]. Indeed, unlike in adults, the incidence and prevalence of asthma in children is higher among boys than among girls, with more exacerbations and more use of emergency services [8]. However, our study did not reveal any gender predominance.

4- Months of hospitalization :

In industrialized countries, an increase in ESA admissions for school-age children has been observed during the first half of September. This is thought to be due to the increased exposure to allergens associated with the start of the school year [12].

Some studies report that changes in global climate play a role in the frequency of attacks, mainly through increased ambient humidity, which increases the risk of exacerbation in asthmatics [13]. Winter predominance was reported in our study, particularly in November, December and January, with a peak in April.

5- **Comorbidities and previous hospitalizations :**

The children in our study had associated pathologies (73%), including allergic rhinitis (23%).

The study by Porcaro et al. highlighted the importance of screening for comorbidities in the context of asthma. Indeed, this finding highlights that the presence of comorbidities favours the frequent occurrence of severe asthma exacerbations by contributing to uncontrolled asthma [14].

6- **Environment :**

There is now increasing talk of the influence of the atmospheric environment on asthma exacerbations in children, and the need for better identification of aggravating factors for optimal management. Firstly, there is the influence of the atmosphere and outdoor pollution [2]. In Milan, Italy, for example, the number of hospital admissions is closely linked to high concentrations of carbon monoxide (CO) and nitrogen dioxide (NO2) [15].

Passive smoking must be systematically investigated during exacerbations.
and contributes to poor asthma control in children [2].

The environment of the Bizerte region is known for exposure to humidity and industrial pollution. In our series, exposure to humidity was the most frequently identified factor, followed by passive smoking.

7- **Asthma :**

7-1- Atopy :

The main virus responsible for exacerbations is rhinovirus, which is thought to cause more severe exacerbations in atopic children [16]. According to several studies, the presence of a recent severe asthmatic exacerbation remains a risk factor &recurrence in the six months following a severe exacerbation in severe asthmatic children aged between six and 11 years [17,18]. In our series, 43% of children with allergy presented with a severe asthma exacerbation, and none of them had a food allergy. What's more, a small percentage of our patients (33%) were already diagnosed with asthma. In this regard, some studies suggest that treatment of allergic rhinitis with nasal corticosteroids improves asthma control in children and may therefore reduce the risk of asthma exacerbation [19].

7-2- History of asthma and level of control :

Non-adherence to asthma therapy is a factor in the occurrence of severe asthma exacerbations [20]. In a study carried out in Morocco, 12% of children had stopped their background treatment in the 3 months preceding the asthma exacerbation [19]. This is consistent with our results, where the majority of our known asthmatic patients were either poorly compliant, or had poorly or partially controlled asthma.

The presence of a recent severe asthmatic exacerbation remains a risk factor 0r recurrence in the six months following a severe exacerbation in severe asthmatic children aged between six and 11 years [2].

On the other hand, several studies have shown that there is no relationship between the severity of asthmatic disease and the occurrence of exacerbations requiring hospitalization or recourse to the emergency department [21,22]. Indeed, in the study by Caroll et al. 55% of children admitted to intensive care for acute severe asthma had intermittent or mild persistent asthma [21]. In the study by Khan et al. inaugural attacks (absence of any previous asthma symptoms) were estimated at 11%.
% of emergency room visits for asthma [23]. In our study, 66% of our
patients were not known to be asthmatic.

Among children with known asthma, more than half (57%) had been hospitalized for an asthma exacerbation, a third in the previous year, and only 27% had optimal asthma control in the month prior to hospitalization [8]. In our series, 60% had been previously hospitalized for asthma exacerbation.

8- **Management of severe asthma exacerbations at home :**

A comparative study of asthma severity and duration of symptoms prior to consultation in Australia, involving a cohort of children and adults, concluded that a delay of more than 6 hours was a risk factor for hospitalization [24].

Early treatment is also a crucial component of management.

In our series, 36% received inhaled BDCA prior to admission and 33% received oral corticosteroids, with an average hospital stay of 13 ±11 hours (1h-48h). This could be explained by the fact that patients are admitted to local hospital or dispensary emergency departments, which already begin early management of exacerbations.

In a study carried out in Morocco, 12% of patients had received bronchodilator treatment alone prior to admission for asthma exacerbation, and 28% had received bronchodilator treatment plus oral corticosteroid therapy [19].

In contrast, the study by Deho et al. reported higher figures, with 95% and 90% respectively [10].

III. **The clinical features of ESA :**

1- **Respiratory signs :**

More specific criteria include a drop in SpO_2 , a decrease in vesicular murmur, slurred speech and respiratory muscle activation. Clinical signs of hypercapnia should also be sought, but are rarely present [2]. In our study, sixty percent of our patients had intense signs of struggle, 20% were in the exhaustion stage and 20% had moderate signs of struggle.

2- **neurological manifestations :**

Neurological disorders such as agitation, confusion and coma are signs of severity requiring immediate management [10]. These disorders may require immediate transfer to intensive care with artificial ventilation.

Thirty percent of our patients had consciousness disorders: agitation in 6 cases (20%) and confusion in three cases (10%), with a Glasgow score between 13 and 14/15.

IV. **Para-clinical features of ESA :**

Gasometry is an essential component of any ESA. Capnia (PaCO2) and partial oxygen pressure (PaO2) are part of the criteria used to classify the severity of an exacerbation: a PaCO2 value > 42mmHg or a PaO2 value < 60mmHg classifies the attack as severe [25].

In our study, only one patient presented with PaO2<60mmHg. Mean capnia was 36±8mmHg (22-52) and mean pH was 7.3 (7.2-7.4).

Data on the bacteriological work-up in childhood ESA are limited in the literature. In the Netherlands, a prospective comparative study concluded that the presence of one or more viruses in the RT-PCR was not a risk factor for ESA in children [26].

Chest X-rays are an essential adjunct to the diagnosis of asthma. However, it is not always essential to the diagnosis of ESA.

Various studies report that chest radiography is essential to rule out differential diagnoses and to look for ventilatory disorders such as pneumothorax, pneumo-mediastinum and atelectasis [27,28].

In our series, chest radiography was performed in all patients. Ventilatory disorders such as atelectasis, pneumomediastinum and pneumothorax were found in 36% of cases.

V. **Therapeutic management of ESA :**

1- **Bronchodilator treatment :**

The management of asthma exacerbations in hospital is well codified. Nebulized salbutamol, corticosteroids and on-demand oxygen therapy are the mainstays of treatment in our setting [19]. In the Netherlands, a prospective, analytic multicenter study reported that all patients admitted to a general pediatric ward received salbutamol nebulizations [29].in our series, all patients received terbutaline nebulizations at a dose of 0.15 mg/kg/nebulization, with nebulizations every 15 to 20 minutes. Inhaled anticholinergics were used in 27 patients (90%), discontinuously in all, at a dose of 0.25mg/nebulizer/8h.

A Spanish study published in 2011 reported that all patients with severe asthma exacerbations received inhaled anticholinergics every 2 hours [11].

Injectable BDCA can be used subcutaneously or intravenously in the intensive care setting [27]. This is a second-line treatment to be used if there is no response to inhaled therapy [30]. None of our patients received intravenous salbutamol.

2- **Corticoids :**

Several studies have reported that early administration of systemic corticosteroids on admission reduces the length of hospital stay [29,31,32]. All our patients were treated with intravenous corticosteroids.

3- **Magnesium sulfate :**

Magnesium sulfate was administered in 70% of cases, at a dose of 50 mg/kg over 20 minutes. Several studies report no benefit fornebulized magnesium sulfate in asthma exacerbations in children, compared with conventional treatment, as in the series by Turker et al. or Colin Powell; this is consistent with a study carried out in Morocco [33].

4- **Respiratory assistance :**

The majority of our patients (83%) received oxygen therapy via single nasal cannula or single mask. Non-invasive ventilation, in the form of high-flow oxygen therapy (HFO), was used in 5 patients (16%).

A 2011 study by Mayordomo-colunga et al. concluded that non-invasive ventilation is a ventilatory option for severe asthma exacerbations. However, close monitoring is required to detect failures and complications at an early stage [11].

5- **Hemodynamic support :**

Four patients required hemodynamic support, including vascular filling. Two were also treated with vasoactive drugs.

The study by Deho et al. reported hemodynamic disturbances in 14 patients. Most required filling without the use of vasoactive drugs [10].

6- **Antibiotic treatment :**

The rate of bacterial superinfection is notable in the paediatric population, and isolation of the causative germ is not easy in respiratory infections. This was also observed in the prospective multicenter study carried out in the Netherlands, with similar results [30]. The percentage of patients admitted for ESA who received antibiotic therapy was 41% [29].

VI. **ESA evolution and mortality :**

1- **Complications :**

Various studies have reported an average hospital stay of between 1.8 and 3.8 days [24,29,34]. Our mean hospital stay is close to those reported in the literature, at 3 ±2 days (0.4-11 days). In our study, we observed 6 cases of atelectasis, 4 cases of pneumomediastinum and one case of pneumothorax. The study by Deho et al. reported one case of pneumothorax [10].

It has been reported in the literature that a visual dyspnea assessment scale, more effective than FeNO or FEV1 in predicting relapse, has been developed for children hospitalized for asthma attacks from the age of six [35]. Programs to support children after an exacerbation reduce the risk of relapse and improve quality of life [2].

Side effects of BDCA can also occur as complications, such as hypokalemia and hyperglycemia [36]. In our study, hypokalemia accounted for 26% and hyperglycemia 6%.

2- **Mortality :**

Mortality was higher in series performed in intensive care units, where patients are more severe. No deaths were recorded in our study. In their multicenter retrospective study of 590 patients in Dutch intensive care units, Boeschoten et al. reported a mortality rate of 0.6% [26].

Conclusions

Severe asthma exacerbations (SAEs) are characterized by a significant deterioration in the patient's usual state of health, as well as failure to respond to well-administered medical treatment, which can be life-threatening and require immediate attention.

It is therefore imperative to identify children at risk of severe asthma exacerbations. Early management of these cases is crucial, to prevent recourse to mechanical ventilation and improve the overall prognosis of the disease.

We conducted a retrospective, longitudinal and descriptive study in the
in the pediatrics department of Bizerte University Hospital.

This study included all children aged under 15 hospitalized for severe asthma exacerbations over a period of 1 year and 6 months (between January 1, 2022 and June 30, 2023).

The aim of our study was to investigate the clinical, para-clinical, therapeutic and evolutionary characteristics of patients hospitalized for ESA in a general pediatric ward.

Demographic, clinical, para-clinical, therapeutic and evolutionary data were extracted from medical records.

Thirty patients were identified, with an incidence of 0.7 new cases of ESA/100 hospitalizations in the pediatric ward. The mean age was 47±30 months (10-132 months), with a gender ratio of 1. Comorbidity was noted in 73% of cases. Peak admissions were in April (20%). Thirteen patients (43%) had associated allergic manifestations, and no patient presented with a food allergy. Ten patients (33%) were known asthmatics undergoing background treatment. Six patients (60%) had been previously hospitalized for asthma exacerbation. The mean time to hospital was approximately 13±11 hours (1-48 hours). Prior to hospitalization, inhaled BDCAs were used in 11 cases (36%). Ten patients (33%) received an oral corticosteroid dose of 1 mg/kg.

Clinical examination on admission showed a mean respiratory rate of 52±10 cycles/minute (40-78), a mean SpO2 of around 91±2% (82-95) on room air. Sixty percent of our patients had shown signs of intense struggle, 20% were in the exhaustion stage and 20% had moderate signs of struggle. Seventeen children were cyanotic and covered in sweat (56%).

Pulmonary auscultation revealed auscultatory silence in 1 case (3%). Slurred speech was noted in fourteen patients (46%). Four patients went into shock. On the neurological level, 30% of our patients presented disorders of consciousness. With regard to arterial gasometry, the mean pH was 7.3 (7.2-7.4) and the mean capnia was 36 ±8 mm Hg (22-52).

Biologically, hyponatremia was observed in three cases (10%). Hypokalemia was noted in 2 cases (6%). CRP above 50mg/l was observed in 5 patients. Chest X-rays showed bilateral pulmonary distension in all patients, associated with ventilatory disorders in 34% of cases.

Bacterial superinfection was confirmed by positive blood cultures in two
patients. The germ was ampicillin-sensitive Streptococcus pneumoniae.

Therapeutically, all our patients received intermittent nebulizations of terbutaline. Nebulized inhaled anticholinergics were administered in 27 patients (90%). Intravenous corticosteroids were administered to all our patients. The molecule used was methylprednisolone (Solumedrol). The prescription rate for magnesium sulfate was 50%. In our study, conventional oxygen therapy was predominant (83%). High-flow oxygen therapy (HFO) was used in 5 patients (16%). None of our patients were intubated.

Complications were mainly ventilatory disorders, such as atelectasis, and high blood sugar levels. The outcome was favorable in all cases.

The results found in our study were partly consistent with the literature. Indeed, several studies showed a male predominance. Some studies found an age of over 3 years. Various series found clinical signs of altered respiratory status with a stable hemodynamic state. Initial gasometry was a criterion for classifying te severity of severe asthma exacerbations. No deaths were reported in our study.

In the light of our results, and based on data in the literature, we can conclude that children aged between 3 and 6 are more prone to severe asthma exacerbations. Asthma exacerbations in children are a seasonal climatic phenomenon for pediatricians. Poorly controlled or uncontrolled asthma, poor compliance with treatment and inadequate specialized follow-up of asthmatic disease are risk factors for severe asthma exacerbations.

Early management by the family remains a key factor in preventing exacerbations, thanks to pediatric diagnosis and support, with specific physiological and developmental features for each age group. Various studies show that predicting the occurrence of an exacerbation is difficult. They do stress the importance of ensuring that asthma control is achieved after an exacerbation, implying that the child should be systematically reviewed one month after an exacerbation [2].

The development of a national protocol for the management of ESA, and the widespread use of high-flow oxygen spectacles in general paediatric wards, has undoubtedly led to improved management.

A multi-center study with a nationwide assessment of the current situation would be of great help in deciding on national recommendations specific to Tunisian children.

References

1.   Global Initiative for Asthma. Global strategy for asthma management and prevention updated 2017 [Online]. May 2017 [Accessed 26 Dec 2023]. Available from URL: https://ginasthma.org/

2.   Carsin A, Pham Thi N. Exacerbations asthmatiques : spécificités pédiatriques (en dehors du traitement). Rev Mal Respir. Dec 2011;28(10):1322-8.

3.   Delmas MC, Fuhrman C.   Asthma in France: summary of data descriptive epidemiology. Rev Mal Respir. Feb 2010;27(2):151-9.

4.   Bouayad Z, Afif H. Epidemiology of asthma and rhinitis in developing countries. Southern Mediterranean. Rev Fr Allergol Immunol Clin. Jan 1998;38(7):154-9.

5.   Hernández Garduño E. Asthma mortality among Mexican children: rural and urban comparison and trends, 1999-2016. Pediatr Pulmonol. 2020 Apr;55(4):874-81.

6.   Zmantar I. Severe asthma exacerbation in pediatric intensive care: clinical, therapeutic and evolutionary aspects [dissertation: medicine]. Tunis: Université de Tunis El Manar; 2022.

7.   Pilar J, Alapont MV, Lopez Fernandez YM, Lopez Macias O, Garcia Urabayen D, Amores Hernandez I. High-flow nasal cannula therapy versus non-invasive ventilation in children with severe acute asthma exacerbation: an observational cohort study. Med Intensiva. 2017 Oct;41(7):418-24.

8.   Fuhrman C, Delacourt C, De Blic J, Dubus JC, Thumerelle C, Marguet C, et al. Characteristics of hospitalizations for asthma exacerbation in pediatrics. Arch Pediatr. Apr 2010;17(4):366-72.

9.   Rampa S, Allareddy V, Asad R, Nalliah RP, Allareddy V, Rotta AT. Outcomes of invasive mechanical ventilation in children and adolescents hospitalized due to status asthmaticus in United States: a population based study. J Asthma. 2015 May;52(4):423-30.

10.   Deho A, Lutman D, Montgomery M, Petros A, Ramnarayan P. Emergency management of children with acute severe asthma requiring transfer to intensive care. Emerg Med J. 2010 Nov;27(11):834-7.

11.   Mayordomo Colunga J, Medina A, Rey C, Concha A, Menéndez S, Arcos ML, et al.

Non-invasive ventilation in pediatric status asthmaticus: a prospective observational study. Pediatr Pulmonol. 2011 Oct;46(10):949-55.

12. Øymar K, Halvorsen T. Emergency presentation and management of acute severe asthma in children. Scand J Trauma Resusc Emerg Med. 2009 Sep;17:40.

13. Mireku N, Wang Y, Ager J, Reddy RC, Baptist AP. Changes in weather and the effects on pediatric asthma exacerbations. Ann Allergy Asthma Immunol. 2009 Sep;103(3):220-4.

14. Porcaro F, Ullmann N, Allegorico A, Di Marco A, Cutrera R. Difficult and severe asthma in children. Children. 2020 Dec 10;7(12):286.

15. Giovannini M, Sala M, Riva E, Radaelli G. Hospital admissions for respiratory conditions in children and outdoor air pollution in southwest Milan, Italy. Acta Paediatr. 2010 Aug;99(8):1180-5.

16. Olenec JP, Kim WK, Lee WM, Vang F, Pappas TE, Salazar LP, et al. Weekly monitoring of children with asthma for infections and illness during common cold seasons. J Allergy Clin Immunol. 2010 May;125(5):1001-6.

17. Haselkorn T, Zeiger RS, Chipps BE, Mink DR, Szefler SJ, Simons FR, et al. Recent asthma exacerbations predict future exacerbations in children with severe or difficult-to-treat asthma. J Allergy Clin Immunol. 2009 Nov;124(5):921-7.

18. Hermosa JLR, Sánchez CB, Rubio MC, Mínguez MM, Walther JS. Factors associated with the control of severe asthma. J Asthma. 2010 Mar;47(2):124-30.

19. Boubkraoui MM, Benbrahim F, Assermouh A, El Hafidi N, Benchekroun S, Mahraou
C. Epidemiological profile and management of asthma exacerbations in children at Rabat Children's Hospital, Morocco. Pan Afr Med J. Mar 2015;20(1):73.

20. Rank MA, Hagan JB, Park MA, Podjasek JC, Samant SA, Volcheck GW, et al. The risk of asthma exacerbation after stopping low-dose inhaled corticosteroids: a systematic review and meta-analysis of randomized controlled trials. J Allergy Clin Immunol. 2013 Mar;131(3):724-9.

21. Carroll CL, Schramm CM, Zucker AR. Severe exacerbations in children with mild asthma: characterizing a pediatric phenotype. J Asthma. 2008 Aug;45(6):513-7.

22. Macias CG, Caviness AC, Sockrider M, Brooks E, Kronfol R, Bartholomew LK, et al. The effect of acute and chronic asthma severity on pediatric emergency department

utilization. Pediatrics. 2006 Apr;117(4):86-95.

23.   Khan MR, O'Meara M, Henry RL. Background severity of asthma in children discharged from the emergency department. J Paediatr Child Health. 2003 Aug;39(6):432-5.

24.   Kelly A, Powell C, Kerr D. Patients with a longer duration of symptoms of acute asthma are more likely to require admission to hospital. Emerg Med. 2002 Jun;14(2):142-5.

25.   Tsou P, Cielo C, Xanthopoulos MS, Wang Y, Kuo P, Tapia IE. Impact of obstructive sleep apnea on assisted ventilation in children with asthma exacerbation. Pediatr Pulmonol. 2021 May;56(5):1103-13.

26.   Boeschoten SA, Buysse CP, Merkus PM, Van Wijngaarden JC, Heisterkamp SJ, De Jongste JC, et al. Children with severe acute asthma admitted to Dutch PICUs: a changing landscape. Pediatr Pulmonol. 2018 Jul;53(7):857-65.

27.   Naiim Habib I, Houdouin V. Asthma i n   children and infants. EMC - Pneumology 2021;32(4):1-11 [Article 6-039-A-65]

28.   De Blic J, Drummond D. Asthma in children and young children. EMC - Pediatrics - Infectious Diseases 2021;41(4):1-18 [Article 4-063-E-10]

29.   Boeschoten SA, Boehmer AL, Merkus PJ, Van Rosmalen J, De Jongste JC, Fraaij PA, et al. Risk factors for intensive care admission in children with severe acute asthma in the Netherlands: a prospective multicentre study. ERJ Open Res. 2020 Aug;6(3):126.

30.   British Thoracic Society. British guideline on the management of asthma quick reference guide [Online]. Oct 2014 [Accessed Dec 26, 2023]. Available from URL:https://www.brit-thoracic.org.uk/document- library/guidelines/asthma/bts-sign-asthma-guideline-quick-reference-guide- 2014/

31.   Bhogal SK, McGillivray D, Bourbeau J, Benedetti A, Bartlett S, Ducharme FM. Early administration of systemic corticosteroids reduces hospital admission rates for children with moderate and severe asthma exacerbation. Ann Emerg Med. 2012 Jul;60(1):84-91.

32.   Kang CM, Wu ET, Wang CC, Lu F, Chiang BL, Yen TA. Bilevel positive airway pressure ventilation efficiently improves respiratory distress in initial hours treating children with severe asthma exacerbation. J Formos Med Assoc. 2020

Sep;119(9):1415-21.

33.   Qach O. L'intérêt de la nébulisation du sulfate de magnésium dans les exacerbations d'asthme chez l'enfant. Rev Fr Allergol. June 2020;60(4):362.

34.   Malmström K, Kaila M, Korhonen K, Dunder T, Nermes M, Klaukka T, et al. Mechanical ventilation in children with severe asthma. Pediatr Pulmonol. 2001 Jun;31(6):405-11.

35.   Khan FI, Reddy RC, Baptist AP. A pediatric dyspnea scale for use in hospitalized patients with asthma. J Allergy Clin Immunol. 2009 Mar;123(3):660-4.

36.   Pardue Jones B, Fleming GM, Otillio JK, Asokan I, Arnold DH. Pediatric acute asthma exacerbations: evaluation and management from emergency department to intensive care unit. J Asthma. 2016 Aug;53(6):607-17.

Appendices

APPENDIX: GINA 2021 assessment of previous treatment level

Children 5 years and younger

Exclude alternative diagnoses
Symptom control & modifiable risk factors
Comorbidities
Inhaler technique & adherence
Parent preferences and goals

Personalized asthma management:
Assess, Adjust, Review response

REVIEW
ASSESS
ADJUST

Symptoms
Exacerbations
Side-effects
Parent satisfaction

Treat modifiable risk factors and comorbidities
Non-pharmacological strategies
Asthma medications
Education & skills training

Asthma medication options:
Adjust treatment up and down for individual child's needs

STEP 1
STEP 2
STEP 3
STEP 4

PREFERRED CONTROLLER CHOICE

Daily low dose inhaled corticosteroid (ICS)
(see table of ICS dose ranges for pre-school children)

Double 'low dose' ICS

Continue controller & refer for specialist assessment

Other controller options

Daily leukotriene receptor antagonist (LTRA), or intermittent short courses of ICS at onset of respiratory illness

Low dose ICS + LTRA
Consider specialist referral

Add LTRA, or increase ICS frequency, or add intermittent ICS

RELIEVER

As-needed short-acting β₂-agonist

CONSIDER THIS STEP FOR CHILDREN WITH:

Infrequent viral wheezing and no or few interval symptoms

Symptom pattern not consistent with asthma but wheezing episodes requiring SABA occur frequently, e.g. ≥3 per year. Give diagnostic trial for 3 months. Consider specialist referral.

Symptom pattern consistent with asthma, and asthma symptoms not well-controlled or ≥3 exacerbations per year.

Asthma diagnosis, and asthma not well-controlled on low dose ICS

Asthma not well-controlled on double ICS

Before stepping up, check for alternative diagnosis, check inhaler skills, review adherence and exposures

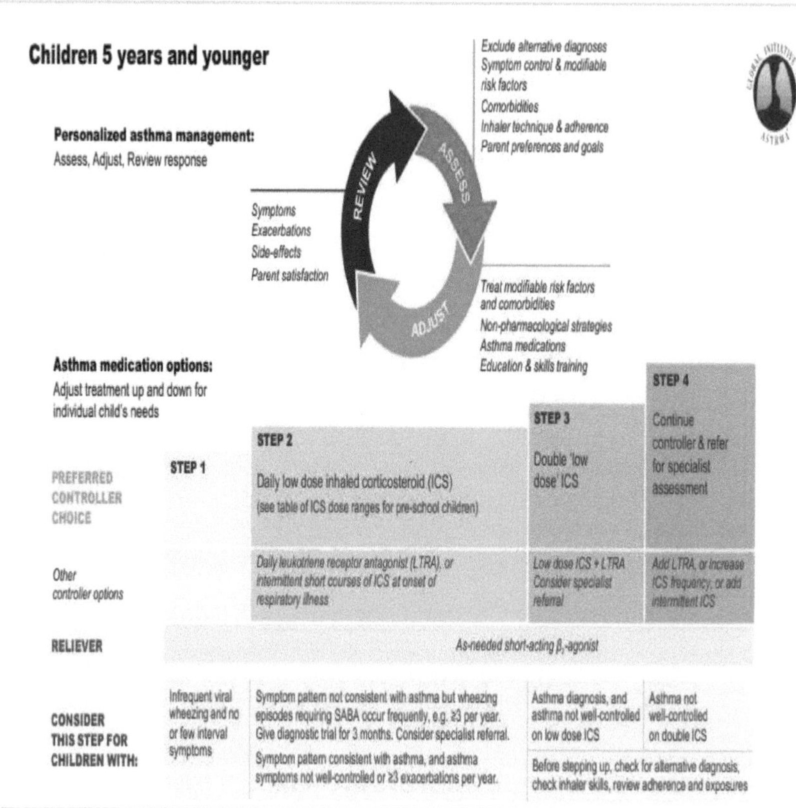

SEVERE EXACERBATION OF ASTHMA IN PEDIATRIC SETTINGS

Abstract

Introduction: Severe asthma exacerbation (ESA) is a change in the patient's usual condition, which also does not respond to well-conducted medical treatment that can be life-threatening and requires urgent treatment. The objective of our study was to study the clinical, paraclinical, therapeutic and progressive characteristics of ESA in a pediatric department.

Methods: This is a retrospective, longitudinal and descriptive study, carried out within the pediatric department of the university hospital of Bizerte, which included children hospitalized for ESA, during a period of 1 year and 6 months.

Results: Thirty patients were identified. The average age was 47 months (10-132 months) with 43% between 3 and 6 years old. Atopy was found in 43% (n=13). Six patients were previously hospitalized for asthma exacerbation. The average hospitalization time was 13

±11hours (1-48 hours). The clinical severity criteria found were signs of intense respiratory struggle in 60% of cases, with auscultatory silence in 3% of cases (n=1), speech disorders in 46% of cases (n=14) and 30% of patients had impaired consciousness. The average respiratory rate was 52 ±10 cycles/minute (40-78), the average SpO2 was 91 ±2% (82-95) on room air. On gas analysis, the mean pH was 7.3 (7.2-7.4) and the mean capnia was 36

±8 mm Hg (22-52). Biologically, hyponatremia was observed in 10% of cases (n=3). Hypokalemia was noted in 6% cases (n=2).

Ventilatory disorders were noted in 36% of cases (n=11). Therapeutic management was based on terbutaline nebulizations, combined with anticholinergics in 90% of patients (n=27) with intravenous corticosteroid therapy. Magnesium sulfate was administered in 70% children (n=21). Conventional oxygen therapy was necessary in 83% of cases with recourse to high flow oxygen therapy (OHD) in 5 patients (16%).

Conclusions: Strengthening therapeutic education for parents of asthmatic children represents a pillar of preventive management of these severe exacerbations.

Keywords: "Child", "asthma attack", "disease exacerbation", "management".

SEVERE ASTHMA EXACERBATION IN THE PEDIATRIC SETTING

Summary

Introduction: A severe asthma exacerbation (SAE) is a change in the patient's usual state of health, which is also unresponsive to well-managed medical treatment, may be life-threatening and requires urgent treatment. The aim of our study was to investigate the clinical, para-clinical, therapeutic and evolutionary characteristics of ESAs in a paediatric ward.

Methods: This was a retrospective, longitudinal, descriptive study conducted in the pediatrics department of Bizerte University Hospital, which included children hospitalized for ESA over a period of 1 year and 6 months.

Results: Thirty patients were enrolled. Mean age was 47 months (10-132 months), with 43% between 3 and 6 years of age. Atopy was present in 43% (n=13). Six patients had been previously hospitalized for asthma exacerbation. The average hospital stay was 13 ±11 hours (1-48 hours). Clinical severity criteria were signs of intense respiratory struggle in 60% of cases, with auscultatory silence in 3% (n=1), slurred speech in 46% (n=14), and impaired consciousness in 30%. Mean respiratory rate was 52 ±10 cycles/minute (40-78), mean SpO2 91 ±2% (82-95) in room air. Gasometry showed a mean pH of 7.3 (7.2-7.4) and a mean capnia of 36 ±8mmHg (22-52). Biologically, hyponatremia was observed in 10% of cases (n=3). Hypokalemia was noted in 6% (n=2). Ventilatory disorders were noted in 36% of cases (n=11). Therapeutic management was based on nebulized terbutaline, associated with anticholinergics in 90% of patients (n=27), with intravenous corticosteroid therapy. Magnesium sulfate was administered in 70% of children (n=21). Conventional oxygen therapy was required in 83.3% of cases, with high-flow oxygen therapy (HFO) used in 5 patients (16%).

Conclusions: More therapeutic education for children's parents is a key factor in the preventive management of these severe exacerbations.

Key words: "Child", "asthma attack", "disease exacerbation", "management".

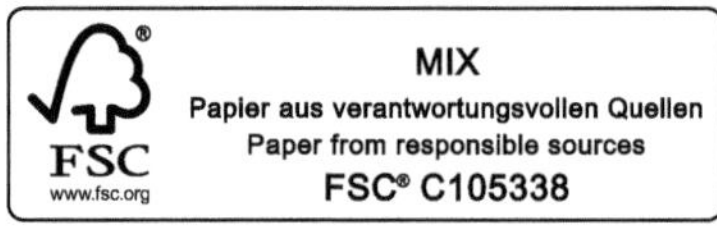

Printed by Books on Demand GmbH, Norderstedt / Germany